ON PRESERVATION

OF

HEALTH IN INDIA

Owing to the antiquity and rarity of this book, certain pages are regrettably absent, and readability is compromised due to the blurring of the original text. If you possess any insights regarding the availability of these missing sections, kindly inform us. Your assistance is crucial in ensuring the completion of this significant work for the benefit of future generations.

ON PRESERVATION

OF

HEALTH IN INDIA.

BY

J. FAYRER

GYAN

Published by

Gyan Publishing House
5, Ansari Road
Daryaganj, New Delhi-110002
Phone: 011-47034999, 9811692060
E-mail: books@gyanbooks.com

Distribution Network
gyanbooks.com
India, USA, Canada, UK, Australia

ISBN: 978-93-6433-474-7 (PB)
First Published, 1894

2nd Impression 2024

Printed at: Gyan Press, Delhi.

ON PRESERVATION OF HEALTH IN INDIA
Author: J. FAYRER

ON PRESERVATION
OF
HEALTH IN INDIA

ON PRESERVATION

OF

HEALTH IN INDIA

BY

SIR J. FAYRER, K.C.S.I., M.D. F.R.S.

PRESIDENT OF MEDICAL BOARD AT THE INDIA OFFICE

London

MACMILLAN AND CO.

AND NEW YORK

1894

PREFACE

THE following pages contain the substance of a lecture delivered to the students of the Cooper's Hill College, as a guide towards the preservation of health in India.

Being now out of print, the author has thought its reproduction in the present form may be useful to those—especially the young—who are about to spend part of their life in India.

ON PRESERVATION OF HEALTH IN INDIA

FEW people who have not been there appreciate the importance or realise the vastness of British India. That extensive portion of the British dominions is the great central and southern promontory of Asia, lying between the 6th and 35th parallels of north latitude, and the 66th and 104th meridians of east longitude (including Burmah and the Shan States). It includes a portion of Afghanistan in the north-west, and part of the country on the eastern side of the Bay of Bengal, extending to Tenasserim, as far south as the 10th parallel of north latitude, and has a coast-line of approximately 4,600 miles. It is about 1,900 miles from Peshawar to Cape Comorin, and about the same distance from Sudya, a frontier point in Assam, to Kurrachi, at the mouth of the Indus;

from Bombay to Point Palmyras, in Orissa, it is 900 miles. The superficial area is above 1,600,000 square miles—nearly equal to the whole of Europe, excluding Russia—and three fifths are directly under British rule.

The geographical boundaries are well defined on the north by the Himalayas, a chain of stupendous mountains, 150 miles in average breadth, the highest in the world, running north-west and south-east in a crescentic manner for 1,600 miles, with a mean height of 16,000 to 20,000 ft., Mount Everest and Kinchinjunga, the loftiest peaks, being 29,000 and 28,000 ft. above sea-level. This barrier, which separates India from Turkestan and Thibet, is crossed by passes up to 17,000 ft. above the sea-level, nearly as high as the line of eternal snow.

On the north-west it is bounded by the edge of the plateau of Afghanistan and Baluchistan, and by the Sulaiman and other mountain ranges; on the north-east by the heights of Assam, dividing the drainage of the Brahmaputra from that of the Irrawaddy. It has the Bay of Bengal on the east, and the Indian Ocean and Arabian Sea on the west.

This extensive but compact country has two hundred and eighty-nine millions of inhabitants, composed of races more numerous and ethnically distinct, and speaking languages more varied, than those of Europe; whilst, from the nature of its physical geography and the extent of its area, it has every kind of climate, varying from that of the torrid to the arctic zone. The seat of a most ancient civilisation, with a history that reaches far back into remote antiquity; possessing a fertile soil, lofty mountains, elevated table-lands, rich alluvial valleys, vast desert tracts and plains, noble rivers, extensive swamps, jungles, and magnificent forests, a rich fauna and flora, wealth of mineral, vegetable, and animal products, and many undeveloped resources, it has characters that invest it with peculiar interest, especially for those who have to reside there.

A country with such physical characters has many distinguishing features of climate that are strange to the European, who has necessarily much to learn before he is acclimatised and adapted to his new home. The people and their habits, the animal and vegetable creation, even the diseases differ from those he has hitherto known, and he makes acquaintance—let us hope not in his own person—with malarial and liver disease, insolation, dysentery, cholera, and others, that at times sweep over the country as destructive epidemics, whilst the conditions of life generally under which he exists differ from those of more northern regions.

This is a field that has, as yet, been only partially explored, but which offers prospect of a rich return to those who work in it. Now, to be enabled to take advantage of this, health is essential, and, though more precarious than at home, it is not necessarily so seriously imperilled as might be supposed, if only ordinary precautions be taken to preserve it.

As having an important hygienic bearing on the subject, a few words may be said on the climate, seasons, and some other matters that affect the health of Europeans generally in India.

The Englishman has naturally a great power of adapting himself to altered conditions of existence, to extremes of temperature and climatic change. Like some of the domestic animals he takes with him, he exists, nay thrives, among the ice of the polar regions, or under the vertical sun of the torrid zone. This power of endurance is often severely taxed, though the strain is sometimes due more to himself than to his surroundings; still there can be no question that, with care, his toleration may be much enhanced. It is reported of an Irish soldier that he said, in reference to the evil effects of climate on his comrades—"They eat and they drink, and they drink and they eat, till they die, and then they write home and say it was the climate that killed them." The soldier was not so far wrong in his estimate of the part climate plays, though he put it *more hibernico.*

In these days of expeditious travelling, men are transported rapidly from one extreme to the other. The sudden change is itself a severe trial, and, if incautiously undertaken, may lay the foundation of a chronic intolerance of the climate.

It is very desirable that Indian life should commence if possible in the cold season, for which reason it is advisable to leave England in October, so as to arrive early in November. Thus there will be no excessive heat on the passage out, and residence in India will begin under favourable auspices, for the cold season will form a fitting preparation for the heat that is to come.

A young Englishman starting with fair health, good habits, and freedom from tendency to organic disease may hope to live well and happily, find scope for the full development and exercise of his physical and intellectual energies, and return to England after long residence in India, able to enjoy life and to work as well as others of his own age, but probably not half his experience. This, however, will depend very much on how he has adapted himself to the varying conditions of life to which he is exposed.

India, in regard to climate, may be divided as follows :—

1. The Himalayan region, with Bhotan, Nepal, Guhrwal, and Cashmere.

2. The Indo-Gangetic plain, or Hindustan proper, which extends along the foot of the Himalayan range, and includes the alluvial plains of the great rivers Brahmaputra, Ganges, and Indus, with their numerous tributaries; the most fertile and important part of the whole empire. The provinces included in this region are Bengal, Assam, North-Western Provinces, Oude, the Punjab, Sind, Rajputana, and other feudatory States.

3. Peninsular India, the Deccan, which consists of elevated plateaux from 1,500 to 3,000 feet above the sea-level, littoral plains intersected by numerous rivers, mountain ranges, and isolated hills. The Vindyah chain, covered with forest vegetation, and its offset, the Satpurahs, traverse the continent from the Western to the Eastern Ghauts (the former rising from 3,000 to 7,000 feet), which bound it on either coast. The provinces included in Peninsular India are the Central Provinces, Berar, Madras, Bombay, Mysore, with the territories of the Nizam, Scindia, Holkar, and other feudatory States.

The climates of this vast territory correspond to latitude, elevation, and physical characters of the country. Northern India is extra-tropical and less influenced than the Deccan by the periodic winds which bring moisture more or less to the whole peninsula. In the former region the climate may be nearly as good as any in Europe; elsewhere it may seem barely compatible with life. Heat alone, however, is not the only objection, for almost everywhere there is added malaria, with the effects of which all, sooner or later, are only too familiar. It is the cause of more sickness and invaliding than almost all other diseases combined, and seldom entirely ceases to manifest its effects on the constitution. Life is maintained under more or less of a struggle, and the object of this paper is to show how the contest may be successfully maintained.

The heat is greatly modified by moisture, the effects of a dry or damp atmosphere at the same temperature being very different. Dry air in motion at the temperature of 100° F. is more tolerable than that at 75° or 80° when stagnant and loaded with moisture. The hot winds of Northern India are more endurable and often healthier than the cooler but humid atmosphere of Lower Bengal or parts of Southern India. Varieties of climate need corresponding adaptation of modes of living, as will sooner or later be learned by experience.

The mean temperatures of the following stations are :—

Calcutta, 21 ft. above sea-level, is in May (hottest month) 85°; January, 65°; but it ranges between 48° in the coldest to 102° in the hottest months.

Madras, 22 ft. above sea-level; June (hottest month), 88°; January, 76°; range, 60° to 108°.

Bombay, 37 ft. above sea-level; May (hottest), 85°; January, 74°; range, 61° to 95°.

Peshawar, 1,110 ft. above sea-level; June and July (hottest), 89°; January, 50°: range, 29° to 115°.

Bangalore, 2,981 feet above sea-level; April (hottest), 80°; January, 67°; range, 51° to 98°.

Poona, 1,849 feet above sea-level; April (hottest), 86°; January, 72°; range, 44° to 106°.

Belgaum, 2,550 feet above sea-level; April (hottest), 81°; August, 70°; December, 71°; range, 51° to 102°.

Lahore, 732 feet above sea-level; June (hottest), 93°; January, 54°; range, 34° to 117°.[1]

The coldest months are December and January; the hottest, April, May, and June.

There are fluctuations in temperature owing to hot dry winds, sea, and mountain breezes, which give local peculiarities of climate. But it may be said generally that there are three distinct seasons

[1] H. F. Blanford, *Climates and Weather of India, Ceylon, and Burmah.*

in India—the hot, the rainy, and the cold, which vary in character according to latitude and elevation, and also in time of setting in and duration; but approximately the cold season extends from November to March, the hot from March to June or July, and the rainy season from that to October. They do not pass abruptly into each other; between each there is a transitional period.

The seasons are greatly influenced in their course and regularity by the monsoons.

The south-west monsoon commences with storms of thunder and wind on the Malabar coast in May, and reaches regions farther north later in the year. The Carnatic and Coromandel coasts, sheltered by the Western Ghauts, are then comparatively exempt from rain.

About Delhi and in the north-west it begins towards the end of June, and the rainfall is greatly diminished. In the Punjab, near the hills, the rainfall increases, but in the Southern Punjab and in the great desert regions there is very little rainfall. There are belts or tracts of country with a rainfall varying from two inches up to some hundreds, the highest being at Cherra Punji, where 600 inches fall; next to this, the Western Ghauts have the greatest rainfall, at Mahableshwar, 263·8 inches; on the Tenasserim coast, on the east side of the Bay of Bengal, it is 180 inches.

In places near the sea, where the land is low and the temperature high, very little rain falls, as in some parts of Sind, where it is under 2 inches; or at Kurrachi, where it is 7·8 inches in the year. In inland districts, where the monsoon has lost much of its moisture, as at Peshawar, only 13·5 inches fall. The rainfall in Calcutta is 65·6 inches; in Madras, 49·1 inches; in Bombay, 74·4 inches; in Delhi, 27·6 inches; in Meerut, 28·5 inches; in Mooltan, 8·3 inches; in Benares, 39·6 inches; in Bellary, 17·6 inches; in Bangalore, 35·6 inches; in Poona, 28·3 inches; in Belgaum, 48·8 inches; in Kamptee, 44·9 inches.[1]

The amount of humidity in the air varies greatly. Some of the lower mountain ranges, Bengal, and many districts near the coast in Southern India are very damp. The elevated table-lands of the Deccan and Central India, and the hot sandy plains of North-West India, have a dry air, and during the months of May and June in the latter it blows like a furnace blast, being heated and desiccated by the hot plains over which it has passed.

The north-east monsoon commences in October, and is attended with dry weather throughout the Peninsula generally, except on the Coromandel coast, where it brings rain from the Bay of Bengal,

[1] Blanford, *op. cit.*

over which it blows between October and December.

In the hill stations of Darjiling, Missuri, Nainital, Murree, Simla, and generally in the elevated provinces of the lower ranges of the Himalayas, also at Utacamand, Kunur, Wellington, Mahableshwar, in the Neilgherries and Ghauts, stations at elevations of 5,000 to 7,000 ft., Europeans enjoy a climate as genial and healthy in summer, and almost as bracing in winter, as in Europe. These are favourite health-resorts, and will probably become the sites of future colonisation, for it seems probable that there the European and his descendants will thrive and continue to reproduce their race; while it is said that after the third generation his progeny would cease to exist in the plains.

The meteorological conditions and physical characters described influence the seasons as follows:—

In Bengal the cold season begins about the middle of October—the days are hot, but the mornings and evenings are cool. The wind is northerly, the air is dry and bracing, the sky bright, though still there may be cloudy days and occasional showers—the last traces of the monsoon. In November and December the weather is cooler, the north-east wind is fresh and sharp, and the air dry;

there are heavy dews at night, dense fogs are apt to prevail, the thermometer ranging from 56° to 78°. About Christmas a few showers occasionally fall. January is colder, the air is bright and keen, fogs are frequent; one may be out all day in the open air, but it is always necessary to protect the head against the sun's rays. The thermometer falls to 46° or lower, and rises to 75° or 76°. Until the middle of February the weather is delightful, but it then begins to get warm at midday. During these months the climate is most agreeable, and those who have been in camp aver that nowhere is there a more healthful and delightful season. It is strengthening to the system exhausted by heat and moisture; the appetite and strength return, and the frame becomes reinvigorated and elastic, but there is risk of visceral congestion, thoracic complaints, bronchitis, &c.

In March the hot weather sets in. The sun is powerful, though the nights are still cool. Atmospheric disturbances, called north-westers, with heavy showers, now cool and freshen the air, and are sometimes accompanied by thunder and hail. Thermometer ranges from 70° to 85°, or higher. In April and May the weather becomes intensely hot, but there are occasional showers and storms that relieve the oppressive state of the air; the skin becomes clammy with perspiration, and irritable from the eruption of prickly heat. The thermometer ranges from 80° to 90°, or higher. The weather is intolerably oppressive, and at nights so close that it is difficult to sleep. The constitution becomes irritable, the nervous system depressed; weakly persons, and especially those who are of intemperate, irregular, or plethoric habits, suffer severely, and not unfrequently succumb to insolation.

There is tendency to fevers and liver complaints. In the commencement of the hot season—February and March—cholera is apt to appear in Calcutta, where, perhaps never quite extinct, its visitations are then most severe. Towards the end of May rain often falls, and is known as the "Chota Bursat," or lesser rains; but frequently the hot muggy weather continues without rain till about the middle of June, when the south-west monsoon sets in with thunder-storms and heavy showers, settling down into heavy rains, which bring the much-longed-for relief, and clothe the earth with verdure; the air is now cooler, but very moist; the winds become variable, and during September, if not before, rain ceases; the air is very damp and oppressive, and it is at this season that the European constitution suffers most; depressed by the previous heat and damp, it is more than ever oppressed by the hot steamy atmosphere in this unhealthy season, when malarious diseases, hepatitis, dysentery, fever, boils, and other torments are apt to occur. During the drying up of the moisture, malaria is active; the vital powers are low, and the constitution is readily affected by it.

In the north-west and Punjab the same sequence is observed, but modified by latitude and physical characters of the country. The cold season is longer, but the sun is powerful, the air dry and bracing, and life in the open air is pleasant. The rains are later, and in some tracts are very scanty, while the hot dry winds in May and June are so intense that the thermometer will rise to 110° or higher in the shade; and were it not for the effect of perspiration, which is free in this parching wind, in cooling the body, life would often be in danger. Indeed, natives as well as Europeans succumb to the "Loo-marna" (hot wind stroke), as it is called in Hindustani. Otherwise, however, it is not unhealthy, and with care a good state of health may be preserved. The heat must be mitigated by the punkah, the tattie, and thermantidote.

In Southern India the climate varies with the peculiar features of physical conformation. The sea-coasts below the Western Ghauts are hot, wet, and steamy; the elevated plateaux are dry or moist according to their proximity to the Western Ghauts. The Carnatic is hot and dry. The thermometer at Madras ranges from 60° to 108°, or higher. The pleasant cold of Bengal and Northern India is unknown there. The ordinary diseases of the tropics prevail, and liver disease is more frequent than in other parts of India. One great compensation, however, it has in its sea-breezes and the proximity to the delightful climate of the Neilgherry Hills.

Bombay is hot and steamy, built on an unhealthy site; but it has been improved, like Calcutta, by sanitary works, whilst its proximity to the elevated plateau of the Deccan and hill stations, its charming scenery, and the sea, make it a favourite place of residence.

Such is a brief sketch of some of the physical characters of India, and of its climate and seasons. This was necessary as introductory to the question of health.

It is now to be considered how to obviate the deleterious action of the climate, and preserve health; what to do in case of disease occurring where medical assistance is not immediately available. The difficulties to be contended against will be chiefly those due to extremes of temperature, dryness, moisture, and miasmata. Heat and cold are relative terms, and people suffer from cold in a hot climate, especially if it be a variable one. The power of tolerating climatic influences is great, if care be taken to observe simple hygienic rules; to avoid exposure to obvious causes of disease; to attend to the nature of the food, drink, clothing, lodging, to take moderate exercise and recreation, and to submit to the moral and physical self-discipline that preserves mind and body in a state of just equilibrium. If the question be asked, how a young man should live with the view to preserve his health in India, the answer is that he should live temperately in all things, always wear woollen, however light, next his person, avoid exposure to the direct rays of the sun, and notoriously miasmatic localities ; go to bed and rise early ; eat moderately, and at regular hours ; smoke and drink as little as possible ; and guard against giving way to passion, excitement, or the irritability of temper so easily acquired in hot climates. He should pay attention immediately to all tendency to bowel complaint or other acute symptoms ; avoid idleness, and its consequent *ennui*, on the one hand, and overwork, mental or physical, on the other. Let him do this, and he may hope to enjoy health, and do his work with advantage to himself and others.

The importance of beginning life in India in the cold season has already been alluded to. From October to February is the best time for arriving (but the nearer October the better), for at all other seasons the Red Sea and the Indian Ocean are so oppressive that he might arrive in India with the seeds of mischief already sown. Of course it may happen to some to have to go at any season ; if so, strict observance of the principles laid down becomes more than ever necessary. It is not asserted that it is impossible to go during the hot, but that it is better to do so in the cold, season.

Suppose a young person to have arrived in India, and to be placed in an isolated position, where he has only himself to rely on, and no one from whom to seek counsel or aid. The first enemy will be the sun, which even during the winter months has great power. He should avoid exposure to it as much as possible between the early morning and the evening hours, but if he must go out, let him wear a good hat made of solah (pith) or other light material, with a puggrie. The head, temples, back of the neck, and spine should be protected. Should he have to be out in the sun in the hot months, let him protect the spine by a pad of cotton, four or five inches broad and twelve or fourteen inches in length. It is well, also, to have an umbrella, which should be covered with white calico to make it more impervious to the sun's rays. During the very hot hours of the day a light pad inside the hat, wetting the puggrie or even the hair, will add to the protection against the heat. Clothing should be light, but not too thin, as a certain amount of substance is desirable to keep out the heat; and light woollen or cotton is the best material.

It is important never, under any circumstances, to omit to wear flannel or light woollen underclothing. This is a cardinal point, and never to be disregarded. The object of wearing it is to equalise temperature and prevent chills. During the action of the skin, the body clothing, if of cotton or linen, becomes wet with perspiration, and the first draught of air that brings it in contact with the person causes a chill, and the evils that may follow are numerous. An extra precaution, sometimes of great value, is the so-called cholera-belt, a band of flannel worn round the body to protect the abdominal viscera from sudden changes of temperature. In many parts of Northern India the cold of winter is severe, and the warmest English clothing is needed. Young men in the vigour of health are apt to neglect and despise these precautions, but they may rest assured that, as matters of personal hygiene, their importance cannot be overestimated, as a few minutes' exposure of the head to a hot sun, the laying aside of underclothing at night because it is hot, may lay the foundation of serious mischief.

Exposure to the direct solar heat, or to a high temperature in the shade, may induce heat exhaustion, ardent fever, heat asphyxia, or other evils of a more insidious character, by injuring the nervous system, increasing irritability, depressing vital energy, and affecting the internal organs, especially the liver, which is already overtaxed by eliminating waste products, and compensating for the diminished respiratory excretion of carbonic acid through the lungs, the consequence of breathing a more rarefied and therefore less oxygenated atmosphere.

In hot climates the blood becomes deteriorated; there is a tendency to liver affections, fever, boils, and a variety of ailments. All are not so affected, for many live for years apparently uninjured by the heat or other climatic influences; but as a rule the European does at length become debilitated, and needs change to a cooler climate, which he should take, if he can, after five or six years. Stimulating or rich food and alcoholic drinks should be avoided, or taken in extreme moderation. Ventilation of dwellings, and especially of sleeping rooms, should be attended to; and, if possible, the latter should be raised above the ground level. It may seem paradoxical to say so, but cold is more to be dreaded at this time than heat, for chills and draughts are most pernicious, and one is never more prone to suffer from them than when bathed in perspiration. A current of air, or the fall of temperature from any cause, and, above all, the neglect of woollen underclothing, may give rise to chill, and fever, liver disease, dysentery, diarrhœa, or rheumatism may be the result. Serious illnesses have been caused by sleeping in a draught, or in the cold air coming from a thermantidote, or from a chill caused by the punkah pulled suddenly after it had been stopped by the coolie falling asleep. It is well to sleep in a light flannel suit, in order to protect oneself from such chills. In the great heat, people sometimes endeavour to get rest by sleeping in the open air, but this is a dangerous practice, unless in very dry climates, and should be deprecated. The punkah is indispensable: it consists of a framework of wood and canvas with a fringe, which is swung backwards and forwards from the ceiling by a rope passing over a pulley, and drawn by a coolie; by putting the air in motion it communicates a feeling of coolness that is very grateful, and indeed without it, in some parts of India, the heat would hardly be endurable.

The thermantidote is a machine through which, by the rotation of a wheel and fans, a current of cooled air is drawn into the room, and, with the tattie, which is a frame filled with khus-khus, a fragrant grass, is much used in the dryer parts of India, where the rapid evaporation of the water sprinkled on the grass produces a great fall in the temperature. For example, in May, in Oude, with a hot west wind, the thermometer stood in shade 104°, in house 83°, behind the tattie, 68°.

The direct action of the sun, or a very high

temperature in a damp atmosphere whether by day or night, in some cases causes very dangerous symptoms, often resulting, after partial recovery, in permanent injury to the nervous system. Those especially who are debilitated or intemperate are in danger, as is often sadly illustrated in the hot oppressive nights of May and June in close rooms, in railway carriages, and the like, in Bengal and other parts of India. In the dryer atmosphere, if the natural refrigerating powers of the body are lowered by disease or intemperance, many succumb during the hot winds, but those who live carefully and take ordinary precautions are in less danger.

With regard to diet, it should be plain and simple: for new arrivals it is better to abstain from much animal or stimulating food, with the view of avoiding plethora, dyspepsia, malassimilation, and congestion of the liver. Moderation is necessary, but it is not expedient to imitate too closely the natives of the country in the character of their food. The stomach of the European will no more obtain from the diet of a Hindoo all that is necessary for nutrition than it could in other circumstances from the blubber that delights whilst it nourishes an Esquimo. Habit, in these things, becomes hereditary, and our machinery is not adapted for sudden changes. But the principle of simplicity is sound, and the food should be modified, to suit changed circumstances.

As a general rule, people eat too much in India —more than they can assimilate, or is needed for nutrition. The consequence is derangements of digestion, faulty assimilation, disordered liver, and engorged portal system, bowel complaints, and the presence of effete matter in excess in the blood. A cup of tea may be taken before the early morning ride or walk; a plain breakfast of tea, coffee, bread and butter, eggs, or even a bit of chicken or fish and rice, at 9 or 10; lunch or tiffin at 1 or 2 P.M., with very little animal food, a cutlet or leg of a fowl, or a little curry, with vegetables, will suffice, and a glass of light wine or bitter beer if desired. People generally dine in the evening. This will be the principal meal of the day: it should be a judicious one—the simpler and plainer the dishes the better, with a little light wine or weak whisky-and-water. The good old maxim of "leave off with an appetite" should be borne in mind. It is needless to detail particular articles of food—that may well be left to the discretion; but the importance of being abstemious cannot be too strongly insisted on. As to wine, beer, and spirits, freely admitting there may be circumstances in which they are required, and recognising the fact that a certain quantity is taken with pleasure, and even benefit by some, it is, at the best, an acquired want that does not originally exist in healthy young men, and, whatever may be said on other grounds, it is not as a general rule a necessity. Great moderation in, if not total abstention from, alcoholic stimulants, excepting when they are prescribed by the physician, certainly increases chances of living and thriving in India. Supposing, however, that abstention be impossible, light wine, such as claret or Rhine wine, is preferable to beer or spirits. The last as an ordinary beverage should be avoided as much and as long as possible. The excuse so frequently given of bad water is not a good one: it is not as a rule made better by mixing it with alcohol. If a stimulant be really needed, let it be of the simplest and purest kind, and never, under any pretext, taken before midday.

As to smoking. It may be pleasant, but it is unnecessary. To many, in moderation, it does no injury; but what is moderation? It often disorders the vision and the heart's action, injures the nervous system, interferes with digestion, depresses the mental as well as the physical, and muddles the intellectual powers. If smoking cannot be avoided, let it be of the mildest and best tobacco, and as seldom as possible—only after eating, and not in the early morning, or till after lunch. This view about alcohol and tobacco may not, perhaps, meet general approval, but it is none the less true. It is the result of observation and experience.

The drinking water is a matter of great importance, and no pains should be spared to obtain it pure. Its impurity is the reputed cause of many diseases, and probably none is more potent for evil. A variety of complaints—cholera, fevers, diarrhœa, dysentery, goître, and some others, including certain parasitic diseases—are ascribed to it. Water should always be filtered, and it is well to boil it ; heat dissipates certain impurities, and tends to render others innocuous. An ordinary sand or charcoal filter should be used, and kept scrupulously clean. The sources of water supply are wells, tanks, rivers, and rain : wherever taken, its probable freedom from contamination by organic impurities should be ascertained. Aërated drinks are not always free from impurities, for the water of which they are manufactured may not have been either filtered or boiled. Turbidity, smell, taste, should rouse suspicion, as these indicate the possible presence of noxious substances, though perfect clearness is not a guarantee of purity. It should be free from smell, and ought to be soft, dissolving soap easily ; if not, there are too many lime salts present in it. It should be clear, sparkling, and colourless ; if it is not so, it may be improved by boiling, filtering, and allowing the sediment to settle. Sediment will be deposited by the addition of a little alum, or other astringent. Boiling destroys the activity of organic matter, and the germs of most of the lower forms of life; it deposits lime salts, and so diminishes the hardness. A green tinge suggests the presence of vegetable matter, not necessarily dangerous; a yellow tinge, sewage contamination or peaty matter, sometimes iron—the first dangerous, the latter two not so. It is firmly believed by the natives that the standing waters of pools, jheels, swamps, and tanks in the forests, the Terai, and malarious localities are charged with fever poison in solution, and it is not improbable that they are right. Such water should always be avoided—at all events, till boiled and filtered. Water may be contaminated by lead or other mineral poison, but this impurity is not frequent. Iced water is much drunk in India: the ice comes from America, or is made artificially. It may be drunk freely in the hottest weather with impunity. Indeed, in the great heat it is good, for it tends to keep down the body temperature.

The use of water externally is of the greatest importance in hot climates, for cleanliness and for keeping the action of the skin free and unimpeded. Generally cold bathing in the morning is best; if it causes a pleasant glow and reaction, it is beneficial; if it depresses or causes chill, it may bring on congestion of the internal organs. Generally it will be found to invigorate, and nothing is more refreshing than a mussuck or gurrah of cold water poured over the head and body; either in the early morning or on return from a hard day's work, marching, shooting, riding, or the like. The swimming-bath is also very pleasant—many stations have them Bathing in lakes, tanks, or rivers is not advisable in the heat of the day. Too much bathing should be avoided, and the temperature of the bath must be suited to the idiosyncrasy of each individual. The warm bath will often give great relief in feverish states or other conditions of indisposition, but it is not a good daily habit.

As regards the dwelling, it should be on a raised site, well drained and ventilated, and as far as possible from low, damp, or swampy ground. Bungalows are one-storied buildings, not always constructed with much regard to sanitary requirements, but are frequently the only houses to be obtained. If possible it is well to get one with a second story, and to sleep upstairs. The room should be large —1,200 cubic feet per head is the smallest space consistent with a due supply of air, and it is better to have more; it should have the proper amount of door and window space, but draughts and currents of air should be avoided. At nights, however great the heat, it is well to have a light blanket, and to wear night-clothing of light woollen. The punkah is necessary during hot nights—without it sleep is often impossible. It is very important to have good sleep, for nothing in the hot weather more refreshes or invigorates you. Mosquitoes must be kept off either by a deep fringe to the punkah or by a mosquito-curtain. Early rising is the rule in India. The morning is the time for exercise and fresh air, and it is well to devote an hour or so to walking or riding. Exercise is essential to health, and it is a duty to obtain it. The use of the Indian clubs, which may soon be learnt from the natives, is a good supplement to other exercise; it develops the chest, and gives vigour to the muscular system. Exercise prevents languor and inactivity, and tends to keep off liver congestion and dyspepsia. It should not be overdone, especially during the great heat, as fatigue and exhaustion may predispose to disease. The mind as well as the body should be exercised. Intellectual torpor and stagnation are as much to be dreaded as physical, and nothing is so likely to prevent irregular habits as well-ordered mental occupation. Europeans in India have generally as much, if not more, to do than they can thoroughly do justice to. But people are not always on duty, and it is right that they should have some resource in intellectual exercise and amusement. There is little difficulty in getting books; reading and the study of the native languages, and the cultivation of any accomplishment, such as music or drawing, will fill up leisure time. Those who are the most fully occupied with professional or official work or business often seem to find leisure for the pursuit of intellectual amusements and field sports, which are conducive, when judiciously followed, to the preservation of health. The habit of work grows, and one learns to utilise every spare moment. Physical health is so much influenced by—indeed, I may say dependent on—mental health that the soundness of one often implies that of the other.

The person who leads a well-regulated and fully occupied life, and who submits to self-discipline, is the healthiest and the happiest. Lapse into irregular habits should be carefully guarded against, for they are apt insidiously to obtain an ascendency exceedingly difficult to resist.

At the same time, over-anxiety about health must be avoided. A proper amount of precaution is right, but coddling and anticipating disease is much to be deprecated. Nothing is worse for a man in unhealthy places or in times of epidemic disease than a state of nervous expectancy and apprehension—it is as unwholesome as it is unmanly. The mind should be kept cool and collected, the ordinary rules for preserving health should be observed, and exposure to direct causes of disease avoided; but it is very necessary to be careful about conservancy, and to see that all bath-room refuse and discharges of disease are disinfected or destroyed. There is no need for supposing every headache is sunstroke or apoplexy, every pain in the stomach cholera or dysentery, every twinge in the side liver. Frequently such things are merely transient disturbances, and pass away. Neither undue apprehension nor unnecessary physicking should be allowed to induce real disease, as they may do. There is no greater mistake than to be always dosing for imaginary or even for real complaints, and sufficient real causes for anxiety exist without inventing imaginary ones. A few words on the general characters of some of the principal diseases and hints on what may be done in emergencies may not be out of place, pending the arrival of medical aid.

Few pass a year in India without learning what fever is, and that there are several forms of the disease. There is simple febricula, that lasts for a few days and passes away, perhaps never to return, without doing any injury. Its symptoms are malaise fever, disordered secretions, headache, muscular pains and weakness, loss of appetite; it may be due to the first effects of heat on a constitution not inured to it, to irregularities of diet, and quite probably to malaria. The treatment is simple. Remain at home, take a dose of aperient medicine, cooling drinks, and a light diet; saline diaphoretics during the hot stage, a few grains of quinine after it has passed away. If it do not pass away in a few days, it will require other management. The precise nature of malaria may not be known, but its effects are very familiar to people in India. No part of India is probably quite exempt, though many are better than others. Heat, moisture, vegetable matter, and its putrefactive changes, certain soils or geological formations, seem to determine the intensity of ague or intermittent and remittent fever.

Malaria is most pernicious in certain districts, and where there is dense vegetation, such as in the Terai, it gives rise to what is called jungle fever Marshes, swamps, and submontane belts of forest, or low jungle, where the subsoil water lies near the surface, such as in the Himalayan Terai, are often deadly and uninhabitable for a great part of the year; the worst season everywhere being in the drying-up months, when heat is desiccating the ground, and liberating malaria. Dry arid tracts of land are not exempt, for it is bad enough in many districts where it cannot be attributed to surface moisture; but it may be that subsoil damp is the cause. There is probably no more fertile source of disease than stagnant subsòil water and imperfect drainage. It would appear that cultivation and living on the ground will in time improve its salubrity, but beware of newly disturbed ground, or of clearance of vegetation, for there emanations may arise from which the most pernicious malarial fever may result. An example of the consequences of bad surface drainage, improper distribution, or retention of water is the fever that has been for years depopulating a district (Burdwan) in Bengal. Malarial miasmata are influenced by locality, winds, heat, &c. One is more liable to suffer on the leeside of a swamp, for example, than to windward of it. A belt of trees intervening will protect to a certain extent, and a covering of the slightest gauze, such as a mosquito-curtain, will guard the sleeper at night. It is more potent near the ground than at an elevation, hence it is well to sleep in an upper story, or in a bed raised from the ground. People constantly exposed to malaria become to a certain extent inured to it; but ague or fever are not the only modes in which malaria declares its action. Broken health, anæmia, cachexia, enlarged spleen, neuralgia, are frequent results, and it often happens that persons may be driven away by ill-health from malarious districts who have never had fever, though they may have suffered severely in other ways. Such persons not unfrequently get fever after they leave the district and return to Europe. In cases of malarial anæmia, with enlarged spleen—a common result of fever—a mixture of quinine gr. iij. and sulphate of iron gr. ii., taken two or three times a day for some weeks (keeping the bowels regular) will be of benefit, but nothing demands change of climate more imperatively than this. The fever caused by malaria is known as intermittent, because it comes at intervals in a paroxysmal form, with a cold, a hot, and a sweating stage; according to the intervals at which these recur, it is called quotidian, tertian, quartan; or it may come at irregular and longer intervals.

These distinct intervals are rather the exception than the rule in India. The form it assumes appears to depend on the intensity of the poison and the peculiarity of the constitution, and perhaps of the locality. In some cases it becomes what is called remittent, and in others, assuming a more severe aspect, it passes into a condition like that of typhoid, and is very dangerous. These are the forms generally known as jungle fever.

The treatment is, in the first or cold stage, warm drinks, in the hot stage salines, diaphoretics, and after the hot stage has passed away five-grain doses of quinine every fourth hour, which should be continued for some time, until the physiological effect of the drug is produced, as recognised by deafness and singing in the ears. It is well to take a dose an hour or so before the paroxysm is expected, for it may prevent it altogether.

There are other forms of fever—the enteric, which may, like the disease in Europe, be due to specific contagion from drains, cesspools, fæcal contamination or the like, or it may be a form of climatic disease; the true typhus, relapsing fever and dengue cannot be dealt with in a few brief remarks, though, generally, a modification of the treatment already mentioned would be appropriate to support the strength and allay fever.

Another prevalent complaint is dysentery, known by the intense pain and difficulty with which the bowels act, and the passage of mucus and blood.

This should at once be treated with fifteen or twenty grains of ipecacuanha in water, and repeating it once or twice every three or four hours. This, if done early, will nearly always give relief, and arrest mischief. Only liquid nutriment should be given. Afterwards Dover's powder, five or six grains, twice or thrice a day, with two or three grains of quinine, may be useful; at first, no alcoholic stimulants, hot fomentations, perfect rest in bed, and communication with the nearest medical officer are advisable. Any sudden relaxation of the bowels should at once be arrested by a dose of astringent medicine and ten drops of laudanum. This may have been unnecessary, and a dose of castor-oil afterwards may be needed; but diarrhœa sometimes means incipient cholera, and it is an error, if one at all, on the right side to check it. Cholera is recognised by the vomiting and purging of watery fluid, which goes on rapidly, and soon exhausts the patient; cramps and lividity soon set in, and death may result in a few hours. On the first symptom of diarrhœa, laudanum x. to xx. or chlorodyne xv. to xxx. drops should be taken, and repeated in two or three hours if necessary, or cholera mixture frequently, as directed. Turpentine stupes or mustard poultices should be applied to the abdomen; brandy and iced water in small quantities should be given, and the courage and the strength of the patient should be kept up; he must be kept warm, the limbs and body rubbed with powdered ginger. The nearest medical aid should be summoned without delay. In times of cholera prevalence it is well to avoid taking aperients, especially salines; unripe fruit or indigestible matter are to be avoided, pure water is essential. Fatigue or any exhausting work should be avoided, and the mind kept as free from despondency and alarm as possible. All cholera discharges should be disinfected or destroyed, and prevented from having access to the water. In all cases of diarrhœa, until a medical man can be consulted it is well to live upon milk taken in small doses of four to six ounces frequently, *i.e.* at short intervals.

Apropos of malaria and exposure to heat, a few words may here be said on shooting and hunting, during which risks from both are incurred. Snipe-shooting has much to answer for. It is a common form of sport, and easily obtained in many parts of India. It should be avoided in the hottest part of the day, and altogether in notoriously malarious localities, and when indulged in, the head should be well protected from the sun, wet dress changed as quickly as possible, and certainly before sitting down to a meal. As little alcoholic stimulant as possible should be drunk, and cold tea when shooting is the best beverage. When in jungly and swampy malarious places, it is well to take three or four grains of quinine and some food before starting in the morning. In shooting from the howdah or on foot in the hot weather, which is the season for tigers and big game, the head and spine should be carefully protected. Heavy tiffins, with beer, champagne, brandy and soda, and rich dishes, are as destructive of sport as they are of health. If these precautions are taken, much heat and exposure may be endured with a fair chance of escaping mischief. The exercise is good, and the pursuit of big game is not only most interesting, but it helps to develop physical and mental energies.

A few words about exposure to heat, and its results. It may cause faintness or exhaustion, or more serious effects on the brain and nervous system, inducing excitement, unconsciousness, and, if very severe, death from asphyxia. In the event of an attack, the person should be removed into the shade, tight clothing loosened, and cold water applied to the head; if he be pale and faint, a dash or two of cold water, it may be, will rouse; if the prostration be profound, that or a stimulant may do good, but it should be administered with caution; quiet, rest and the recumbent posture will soon restore, but the sufferer should be taken home, and not exposed again to the heat. If the face be flushed and the skin hot, cold water and ice, if it is at hand, should be applied over the head and body; he should be removed to a cool place, an aperient administered, and the bowels kept open. Perfect rest and quiet should be secured, and if recovery is not complete and rapid, medical aid should be sought. An intense form of fever, with head symptoms, may be the result, which requirès active and prompt treatment of the nature before described in reference to ordinary fever. Of course this is but the merest outline of what should be done, but this much, if done promptly, will be of great service, and may save life. One thing to be guarded against is any attempt to bleed the sufferer. The remedies are ice to the head, cold affusion, perfect rest and quiet in the coolest shelter to be found, and aperient medicine.

A few words about liver disease, which begins most probably by pain in the right side and shoulder, fever, nausea, constipation, and a semi-jaundiced skin. Free purgation, with calomel, compound jalap powder, or sulphate of magnesia, fomentations over the side, and very spare diet, excluding meat and alcohol, will probably give relief, and may stave off inflammation and consequent abscess. In such cases the nearest medical aid must be sought. For ordinary bilious derangements, with foul tongue, nausea, sallow face, eyes tinged with bile, a couple of colocynth pills, and a dose of salts next morning, with abstinence from animal food and stimulants, and avoiding exposure to heat, will generally suffice; but any mode of life should be avoided that may appear to tend to increase the disposition to these attacks, for they may end in congestion—perhaps inflammation—of the liver. As to diarrhœa—if it occur when one is otherwise in good health, and if it seem to be due to any indiscretion in diet, a dose of oil or of Gregory's powder should be taken to expel the peccant matter, a light diet should be adhered to for a few days, and all will be well. Diarrhœa *may* be the precursor of an attack of cholera. If that disease is about, check it at once, for reasons formerly given; if from other causes, simple astringents, such as chalk and catechu, with restricted diet, may be sufficient to remove it. Chronic diarrhœa of the tropics requires change of climate and an exclusive milk diet, but details cannot be entered into here.

In connection with functional derangement of the liver, attention may be called to a condition which not unfrequently depends on it, often amounts to serious disease, and is always a source of trouble and annoyance to the sufferer—hæmorrhoids (piles). These are vascular growths (small tumours) connected with the mucous membrane of the lower bowel, either within the orifice or just external to it. They are of two kinds—the internal and external, and depend on a distended, congested, and varicose state of the hæmorrhoidal blood-vessels and mucous membrane, and are much influenced by the condition of the liver, as the vessels implicated form part of the so-called portal circulation, by which is meant the blood that, flowing through certain veins, enters a large trunk called "Portal," the branches of which are distributed to the liver; the blood brought by it being that from which bile and other products are separated. In certain abnormal states of the liver in which the free circulation of the blood is impeded, congestion of these vessels is apt to result, and to give rise to this troublesome affection.

Whilst small and incipient, they are comparatively harmless, but when they increase in size, as they are apt to do, and when they give rise to mucous discharge and hæmorrhage, from rupture of the distended vessels, they are prejudicial, and should be removed or otherwise actively treated.

The *internal* are generally the most troublesome, but both are liable to fits of congestion, inflammation, and, at times, hæmorrhage.

The loss of a small quantity of blood in this way is often attended with a delusive sense of relief, but this cannot go on long without causing serious mischief to the health. It is best to try and avoid having the affection at all, and the way to do so is to keep the bowels regular, avoid luxurious and slothful habits, take plenty of exercise and a moderate diet, bathe the parts with cold water, and avoid excess of food and stimulants of all kinds.

A sedentary life may have induced this disease: if so, it should be got rid of before going to a hot climate, where it is likely to increase.

In case either external or internal piles should have proceeded so far as to cause pain or hæmorrhage, then rest is imperative; saline aperients should be taken, cold and astringent applications or injection may be required; tannic acid or alum in water, or an ointment made of gall-nuts, should be applied; but as soon as possible the nearest medical aid should be sought. When the swelling and tension are severe, hot fomentations with solution of acetate of lead and opium may give relief.

The frequent losses of blood, even in small quantities, are very prejudicial; they cause anæmia and debility, a blanched and pallid appearance, with breathlessness and exhaustion. This should never be allowed to continue, and it is most probable that an operation for the removal of the growths will be necessary. When from any cause, such as errors of diet or stimulants, cold or wet, the piles become inflamed, a dose of calomel gr. iii., opii gr. i., should be taken, and followed with a dose of castor-oil next morning. The recumbent posture and fomentations should be resorted to.

If the pain and tension are very severe, a leech or two, or puncture of the distended tumour, may be expedient. But in such cases, if possible, medical aid should be got.

For those who have a tendency to the affection, careful living, plain food, regular exercise, the use of some mild laxative, such as confection of pepper or senna, or Ward's paste, sulphur and cream of tartar, rhubarb with ipecacuanha and soda, may be very useful, and the application of the gall ointment already mentioned. The use of the enema of cold water every morning after the action of the bowels is often beneficial.

These precautions, necessary everywhere, are especially so in hot and malarial climates, where there is a natural tendency to liver derangement, and therefore these remarks seem especially applicable to those who are to live in India.

Of course there are many other diseases and accidents to which people in India are liable. But those only have been mentioned in which immediate aid is required before it may be possible to get medical advice.

Snake-bites are very dangerous in India, but happily are very uncommon in Europeans, though twenty thousand natives die yearly from this cause. The venomous snakes of India are the ophiophagus, cobra, bungarus (black or steel-coloured and yellow-banded), Russell's viper, and Echis carinata. There are also some others comparatively rare, and the salt-water snakes, which are all poisonous. The cobra, the krait (Bungarus cæruleus), the

Russell's viper, and the echis viper are the snakes most likely to be met with, and their bites are very deadly.

As soon as possible after a person is bitten by a snake, a ligature of cord should be applied round the limb or part, a few inches above the bite. A piece of stick should be introduced, and the ligature tightened to the utmost by twisting. Another ligature may be applied above the first, and tightened like the other. After the ligature has been applied, scarify across the puncture to the depth of a quarter of an inch with a penknife or other cutting instrument, and let the wounds bleed freely. Apply either a hot iron or live coal to the bottom of these wounds as quickly as possible, or some carbolic or nitric acid. Wash and inject freely into the wound, so that it should permeate the tissues, a solution of permanganate of potash, 10 per cent. If the bite be on a part where a ligature cannot be applied, cut out the part, and inject permanganate of potash and cauterise. Give fifteen drops of liquid ammonia diluted with water immediately, and repeat it every quarter of an hour for three or four doses, or longer, if symptoms of poisoning appear; or give brandy, or other spirit, with an equal quantity of hot water, about an ounce of each (for an adult) at short intervals. Should no symptoms of poisoning appear in half an hour after the application of the ligatures, they may be relaxed. In that time, if the permanganate of potash have been well introduced, any poison there would have been neutralised.

Suction of the wounds may be beneficial, but as it may be dangerous to the operator it cannot be enjoined as a duty. If, notwithstanding, symptoms of poisoning set in and increase, if the patient become faint and sick, depressed or unconscious, apply mustard poultices or liquid ammonia on a cloth over the stomach and heart, continue the stimulants, and keep him warm; but do not shut him up in a hot stifling room—rather leave him in the fresh air. A hypodermic injection of 10 to 15 drops of the liquor strychniæ (B.P.) may be given,[1] which may have to be repeated in twenty minutes or half an hour, according to circumstances. Artificial respiration also may be practised. Do not make him walk about if depressed; rouse him with stimulants, mustard poultices, or ammonia, but let him rest. If the person be first seen some time after the bite has been inflicted, and symptoms of poisoning are present, the same measures are to be resorted to; nothing else can be done. The prostration is sometimes due to

[1] *On Snake Poison: Its Action and its Antidote*, by A. Mueller, M.D.

fear; the bite may have been that of a harmless or exhausted snake, and persons thus bitten will rapidly recover. If poisoned, but, as is frequently the case, slightly, these measures are also the most expedient; if severely poisoned, no others are likely to be more efficacious. People should be warned against nostrums, popular antidotes, and loss of time in seeking for aid. The measures suggested are no doubt severe, and not such as under other circumstances should be entrusted to non-professional persons; but the alternative is so dreadful that, even at the risk of unskilful treatment, it is better that the patient should have this—the only—chance of recovery.

Protection from mosquitoes is afforded by a curtain. The irritation may be allayed by a cooling lotion of goulard; the application of sal-volatile and eau de Cologne may give relief; and it is said that camphor, penny-royal, and lemon juice, if rubbed on the skin, will keep them away—which is best of all.

Centipede and scorpion poisoning are comparatively rare. The pain is severe, and in an unhealthy state of the constitution it might be dangerous; but generally a cooling lotion, or ipecacuanha or ammonia, applied externally, seems to neutralise the action, and allay pain.

In the foregoing sketch attention has been called to some of the most important points concerning health and possible sickness in India. Should the suggestions be attended to and the precautions observed, there is every reason to hope that health may be preserved and life spent profitably.